I0436927

Labor of Love

For those who have labored, loved,
and lost; and are forever changed.

Sandra S Schantz, RN, BSN

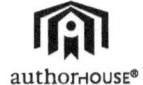

authorHOUSE®

AuthorHouse™
1663 Liberty Drive, Suite 200
Bloomington, IN 47403
www.authorhouse.com
Phone: 1-800-839-8640

© 2007 Sandra S Schantz, RN, BSN. All rights reserved.

No part of this book may be reproduced, stored in
a retrieval system, or transmitted by any means
without the written permission of the author.

First published by AuthorHouse 8/2/2007

ISBN: 978-1-4343-1557-1 (sc)

Library of Congress Control Number: 2007904808

Printed in the United States of America
Bloomington, Indiana

This book is printed on acid-free paper.

This is written for those who have:

labored,

loved,

and

lost.

Labor of Love is dedicated to the babies who left this world too early, leaving us behind to mourn their loss. Their lives, however short they were, have touched and changed us forever.

Mark David Schantz
2/2/70 - 2/5/70
Matthew VanDeuren
6/5/81

Contents

Foreword   ix

Preface Fall 2006   xi

All in a day's work   1

Pregnancy   7

Miscarriage   11

Stillborn and Infant Death   17

Definitions   31

Five Stages of Grief   41

Recovering From Grief and Loss   45

"Coping with Death and Grief"   47

Finding Recovery is a Decision   49

Resources   51

Foreword

"Labor of Love" has indeed been a labor of love for Sandi Schantz, a woman I feel privileged to call my friend and ally in our common goal of pregnancy loss awareness.

I came to know Sandi in 2006 while working on my first book, "Forever Our Angels" and I feel honored to have had Sandi contribute an essay to my second book, "Remembering Our Angels: Personal Stories of Healing from a Pregnancy Loss."

I was inspired by her strength and determination to help grieving parents facing pregnancy, infant and child loss. She is that nurse that a woman wants by her side during the good and not so good times. Her empathy, her compassion, and her support is unparalleled. Sandi truly cares about her patients and she goes above and beyond what is asked of her.

Pregnancy loss continues to be a subject that people feel uncomfortable talking about. My hope is that "Labor of Love" will provide comfort and ease the pain of pregnancy loss.

Foreword contributed by Hannah Stone, Author of "Forever Our Angels" and "Remembering Our Angels: Personal Stories of Healing from a Pregnancy Loss."

Preface

Fall 2006

I was standing at the time clock, waiting for one more minute to pass so I could swipe in. I had my coat on, my purse and lunch bag hung from my left arm as I stood there, my badge ready to swipe, in my right hand.

I noticed a female employee coming down the hall towards me. I didn't recognize her as any of the familiar faces I usually see. (I've worked here for 27 years!) I thought nothing more about it as she slipped into the locker room to put her coat away.

I had my back to the locker room when she came out. I heard someone say, "are you Sandi?" When

I turned to the voice, it was the same woman that I had just seen, but didn't know.

I answered, "yes" while mentally racking my brain for recognition of whom this woman was. I couldn't find anything familiar in the face or voice.

"I just want to thank you for all you did for us when our baby died."

My brain is thinking "your baby died?" I'm looking at a woman probably close to my own age and I'm not at all interested in having babies any more, although technically it would still be possible.

I told her I was glad that I was able to have been of help. I asked her name, and when she told me her name was *Sherry and that her son had died of SIDS, I immediately recalled the situation! I gently asked her how old her son would be now. Without hesitation, she said, "21". I asked if she had any other children because I knew that the son they lost was their first baby. His name was *Michael Ray Jr. She told me she had two more boys, they are 17 & 19 now. I told her I was glad they'd stayed together and had tried again to have a baby.

She then told me she has just started to work at this hospital. As we went our separate ways that morning, to work, I felt so rewarded deep in my soul. Here 21 years later, a mom recognized me! To know that what ever words we shared, pictures we shared, phone calls we shared and tears we shared, touched this woman's life!

Now, when we meet in the hall and smile and say hi, we share something most people probably don't even know about, 21 years after the fact.

All in a day's work

In 1981 I started working in labor and delivery. I was newly married and knew I'd have a family some day. I had worked hard on the orthopedic floor where patients came in for everything from fractured ankles, hips and wrists, road rash from motorcycle accidents (asphalt embedded into thighs and noses shaved off), gangrene of extremities, amputations from gangrene, mowers, saw blades or snow blowers, automobile and train accidents. Some of our patients stayed months at a time. I was ready for a happy job!!!! What could be happier?!!!

Babies are born everyday. Having a baby is a natural part of life. We grow up and have families. Commercials advertise everything from home pregnancy tests, diapers, baby food, Juicy Juice,

1

educational and developmental toys. Working labor and delivery I faced the hearts breaking of families who were forced to face the fact that a pregnancy doesn't guarantee a pink, soft, chubby, cooing baby goes home with them.

In 1982 I was pregnant with my first baby. Labor and delivery is a difficult place to work when you are pregnant. It almost made a hypochondriac out of me. After taking care of someone with a miscarriage, I just knew that unusual feeling I had, would end in a miscarriage. After seeing babies delivered at various stages of pregnancy I would identify my own baby with each of them. When a baby was born with a birth defect I would go home worried that my baby would have a birth defect too. The hardest thing I experienced that pregnancy was having two co-workers that were also pregnant lose their babies.

When I walked into work one afternoon, I saw one of these two nurse's names on our census list. I knew she wasn't due yet. What's going on I wondered. After learning that her baby had died, I went into see her. She was about seven months pregnant. My heart was heavy, my throat constricting and my eyes barely able to hold back my tears as I entered her room. I was surprised to find she was quite composed, being a nurse really, instead of a grieving mom. I remember her saying matter of factly, "**my baby is dead.**" Since the other labor nurses were uncomfortable with an infant death, I took care of them.

Caring for a family in labor with a known stillborn is a very emotionally draining job. Her son was small, but beautiful. The cord had wrapped around his neck five times. I took some pictures of him with a Polaroid camera I found in the nursery. His mom chose not to see him or hold him. She never came for his pictures either. My heart ached for them.

Each day I continued my pregnancy I felt guilty. I couldn't continue to care for those with infant deaths while I was obviously pregnant, for my sake or theirs.

The other nurse I mentioned, *Esther, delivered elsewhere, but I learned she had a full-term stillborn daughter. Her name was *Michelle (Turns out she was the only daughter they would have) She was born in April 1982. Both of these nurses worked in the emergency room. Oh my heart ached for them! How could I help them though, when I had a baby and they didn't?

My own baby was due January 28, 1983. Through out my pregnancy I had prayed that he/she would not be born on January 28th. Why would it matter you ask. There was a couple from our church who had experienced several miscarriages and finally carried a pregnancy to term….plus. They delivered a 12 pound, 4 week over due stillborn son on January 28th, 1982. I didn't want my baby born on the same day as theirs. I didn't want to add to their pain. Thankfully, my son was born February 4, 1983.

As much as I was in love with my son and enjoying his every movement and sound, I kept thinking of those I had worked with and met in the last year who did not have a baby in their arms.

I started reading about pregnancy loss, grief and loss and became a Bereavement Counselor thru Resolve Through Sharing from LaCrosse, WI.

I started keeping records of families experiencing the loss of a pregnancy or baby, due dates and day of death, trying to give follow up calls and letters and cards on the due dates and 1 year anniversary of the death.

*All names used have been used with permission from the families.

Pregnancy

E very one of us who has experienced a pregnancy, whether planned or not, can remember their feelings when they suspected they might be pregnant. Feelings that ranged from excitement, joy, fear and dread.

For those who were excited about being pregnant or accepting of being pregnant, just knowing we were pregnant set a lot of thoughts, events, hopes, plans, and emotions into action.

Most of us can recall where and how we told our spouses, boyfriends, parents, and best friends our news. Some of us made phone calls, wrote notes, or staged a situation with hints. (baby items, baby foods)

From the time we knew we were pregnant, we began planning for this baby. We all have a typical baby image: pink, chubby face, baby blue eyes, toothless smile, the "Gerber Baby" look. Our thoughts fast forward to "What Christmas will be like", 1st birthday, 1st day of school, soccer or softball games, dance, football, first dance, driver's ed, prom, and graduation.

All of these things we think about for a little being, no bigger than a bean, that we don't even know!!

We run through bedroom color schemes and themes, pick up baby name books, and pick up books on "your pregnancy" to read within the first 2-3 months we're pregnant. No one knows we're pregnant yet, unless we've told them. (we're not physically showing we're pregnant yet.)

So…..what happens when we experience a miscarriage?   A stillbirth?   An infant death?

The loss of a pregnancy, a child, is unlike any other death. While the natural order of life would be for parents to be buried by their children, parents burying their children is not a natural, orderly scenario.

When a child, infant dies, it destroys, and steals all the thoughts, emotions, plans, and hopes not only for now, but for all of the future. Parents lose the pregnancy they have now, but also all the dreams for the future, their future, their legacy, and all the dreams for that child.

Miscarriage

*U*sually a miscarriage is defined as a pregnancy that ends (not induced or terminated) of natural causes or injury before the 20th week into the pregnancy. This may vary state to state. This date was chosen because viability outside the womb at 20 weeks or less is very unlikely.

In Indiana, miscarriages do not have to be buried or cremated as do infants that die after 20 weeks of pregnancy. Again, this may vary state to state.

Many times, when a miscarriage is experienced, there isn't a "fetus" (early stages of development of infant) recovered. The developmental stages may be so early, it can't be determined what the sex of the fetus is.

When I did a six weeks follow up phone call to parents having had a miscarriage, the number one question I was asked was, "What did they do with my baby?" The hospital I work at is a Catholic Hospital and I was able to assure my families that "our hospital buries it's miscarriages together in an unmarked grave". When I surveyed the other area hospitals, I found that my hospital was an exception, not the rule re: caring for miscarriages.

The parents experiencing a miscarriage struggle with the fact they were pregnant, and they've lost that baby. Unlike parents who experience a stillbirth or infant death, they weren't able and probably not offered to see their little one. There is no death certificate, no hospital bands, foot prints, lock of hair, obituary or grave. Everyone didn't know they were pregnant, only those they had chosen to tell. No sympathy cards come. Yet, their hopes and dreams for this baby have been stolen and shattered and they have nothing to show for this pregnancy. Sometimes they question their sanity!! "I was pregnant wasn't I?"

When I called one of my patients after her miscarriage, she had really been struggling with identifying her miscarried baby with reality. She had been offered to see her little baby, but opted not to. She now needed some concrete evidence of his existence. With his length and weight and the fact that he was completely formed, she ended up holding and burying one of her other son's GI Joes. That baby was not just an imagination. He was real.

I have found it helpful to give some of my families a detailed, week by week pictorial of developing fetuses, pregnancies, babies. Sometimes our minds do more damage with its imagination. It helps parents to know what they have lost. Sometimes, if the "development weeks" match, I give them a plastic, life size model of a developing baby. Something with which to identify their baby.

I have on occasion, had a teenager, experiencing a miscarriage feel nothing but relief. No one knew, and now, no one will know until she deals with her loss at a later date.

In this day and age, most women experiencing a miscarriage are not seen in the hospital as patients. Often there may be a trip to the emergency room because of cramping or bleeding. There may be an ultrasound done at that time to confirm if the pregnancy is still viable, if there is a heartbeat. If so, the women are told to see their physician for follow up. If there isn't a heart beat and the woman is told, she is still often told to follow up with her physician. Occasionally, if there is no heart beat, the woman might be sent to surgery for a "D&C" which stands for dilation and curettage.

Most often, though, the D&C is scheduled for another day and time. Usually the women are notified of their surgical date and time of arrival to the hospital.

They go through pre-op, surgery, and recovery and are sent home. I don't think there is much support given in the area of pregnancy loss. We tried to get the nurses in recovery to hand out miscarriage booklets to their patients, but they were uncomfortable with that and busy with several patients at once and consequently, I don't think much is done for these families experiencing miscarriage. When they follow up with their doctors, they see the pregnant women in the waiting room. They sit in their chair, waiting their turn. If they're still emotional about their loss, they hope no one asks them about why they are in the doctor's office. They don't want to cry in front of the others in the waiting room.

Miscarriages are not acknowledged as a death. These parents don't have a lot of support because their loss is not treated as a death. I've heard people say, "it was just a miscarriage" "at least you didn't know the baby" "at least you didn't get attached" "at least this happened before you got him or her home." Society doesn't recognize this pregnancy as a hoped for or longed for infant. There are no services, obituary to acknowledge the infant or announce the family's loss.

As with all parents who lose a baby, Mother's day and Father's day are very painful. Especially the first one after the loss. They were expectant parents and they know they would have been good parents.

When the due date comes along, it causes all of the original questions to resurface: "why" "why us" "what if" "if only" and the guilt "what did I do cause this" "what did I do to deserve this?" The "would of" "could of" "should of's" torment their thoughts.

I do encourage my parents of a miscarriage to name their babies. Someday they may choose to tell their other children about this baby. It's easier to refer to a child than just "a pregnancy" They usually will pick a name that could be used for a boy or girl, unless we know what the sex of the baby was. I have given numerous couples a set of small white booties to hang on the Christmas Tree. No one but us knows what those booties stand for and yet it gives them a small way to acknowledge and remember their loss.

Stillborn and Infant Death

When I've worked with families experiencing a stillborn baby, I've found the families really get through labor and or surgery better if they've had a day to adjust to the news and make some plans, some decisions, and then face labor or surgery.

Families are so in shock when told their baby has died that they can't absorb or accept it. "There must be a mistake" "You're wrong" "It can't be". When we immediately force them into labor or surgery, we force them to face what they have not been able to come to terms with. To deliver that baby now, removes all hope that there is a mistake.

I do encourage my families to make as many memories as possible during what little time they have. They need to make memories to last a lifetime. By thinking of it like this, it is not as repulsive to the families to "hold a dead baby". It gives them permission to hold their baby.

I've used a check off list that I would give to the families the day they found out their baby has died. It is my job to prepare them for the next few hours, next few days, and the next few months.

For most young families, having a baby is the first time they've been a patient in a hospital. Most of them still have their parents around. They've not ever had to be involved in planning a funeral. They have no idea what to do first.

When there is time to meet with the family before they get into labor or are whisked off for surgery, I have found it comforting to the families to have some guidance and some control. With the news they've received, everything else is out of their control. I leave the family with this check list and let them talk about it, cry about it, make their own decisions. I've had them just give me the check list when they were done with it, and that check list went with their chart. The decisions have been made, their wishes known and it is up to the staff now, to carry out their wishes. The staff have this list and we now know what they wish to do and not to do. We don't have to ask them again and again. Each shift has that same check off list and knows what the family wants.

I would prepare the family for what would be happening once labor was induced, or a cesarean done. The check list included such things as:

-who do you want here, to see your baby, to share this time with (family, friends, Minister etc)

-Do you want your baby baptized

-Would you like to take pictures of you and the baby, or have pictures taken for you by the staff

-Would you like to remain on the OB unit, or would you like to be on another floor. (If on OB, you might hear babies crying, which will be hard, but you are with nurses who know and care about what's happened).

On another floor, probably your baby, your loss will never be addressed. You'll just be treated like any other medical/surgical patient.

-There will be papers to sign. Do they want an autopsy if the cause of death is not evident. They will have to choose a funeral home for the baby's body to be

released to and sign a paper allowing the baby to be released.

-Would they like the baby to be dressed in a particular outfit to go to the funeral home?

- How about a blanket or stuffed animal?

-Mom needs to be prepared that her body knows she's had a baby (even when it isn't full term) and prepare her for the engorgement of her breasts. If she's had a cesarean, she's had surgery and no baby to show for it.

-Mail will come from anything she's signed up for during her pregnancy.

-Commercials with baby's will bother her (them) People will call (both those who have learned their baby died and those who are just calling to see how the pregnancy is going) They may just want to let the answering machine pick up and be selective as to what calls they answer for a while.

-I warn them of difficult days ahead, Mother's Day, Father's Day, Baby's due date, Christmas, Thanksgiving and the one year anniversary.

I encourage my family to hold their baby, touch their baby, count it's toes and fingers, take pictures of the baby.

As a nurse, it is my responsibility however, to prepare the parents for what their baby may look like, feel like. Sometimes, when parents don't see their baby, they have imaginations that are incredibly wrong, sometimes they might have nightmares of things imagined.

Ultimately, it is the parents choice though and we the medical professionals need to honor their decisions. We take pictures of the baby, both clothed and unclothed.

We don't want imaginations to think we're hiding anything from the parents. Sometimes we'll dress them in clothes the family brings, or we may let the family bathe or dress their baby. Sometimes parents need to love their babies, physically. We keep the pictures for the families. Sometimes they may want them when we follow them up with a phone call, or on the due date or one year later. We have had families that have chosen to not have their baby's picture.

We wrap our babies in a warm blanket, so that our parents hold a warm bundle. We put lotion on the baby's skin and sprinkle a little baby powder in their blanket. The feel of the baby, the warmth of the blanket and the smells of lotion and powder will bring comforting memories to the family down the road....of grief.

Again, it is healthy for families to name their babies, put an obituary in the paper, and have a service of some kind for their baby. An obituary lets people know their baby has died. It makes an announcement and saves the parents from making many painful phone calls.

How many families preparing for a baby are financially prepared for the costs of a funeral and burial? Usually life insurances do not assist with funeral expenses for a stillborn or a newborn infant that dies. There are funeral homes that will do an infant funeral for free or a very minimal charge. As bereavement counselor it's helpful to have the names and phone numbers of area funeral homes available and to know which of them will help with the cost for the family.

If mom has had a cesarean, she needs to be a part of that funeral service. There is no rule or law that says the dead must be buried in three days. The parents are still in shock and the days up to and including the funeral will be a blur of a memory.

I've found it helpful for the funeral to be video taped and given to the family. Even if they never watch it, they have it!

When *Carmen's second baby, and second daughter was stillborn, they named her *Rebecca. I was told instead of having newborn pictures of their infants up on the wall, they chose to put up sets of footprints with each of the girl's names on them.

Some of my mom's have found scrap booking very therapeutic **when** they were ready to go thru the baby's things.

Writing is also helpful and therapeutic. Many keep a diary, write to the baby, and. write poetry.

My young families have not given me positive feed back on Compassionate Friends. They report a lot of time is spent on memories and these young families were robbed of making very many memories in terms of time and years.

Some families find comfort in visiting the grave, others do not. To each his own. There is no right or wrong.

For those families that have survived a pregnancy loss, infant loss and have been able to maintain their "couple" or "married" relationship, I want to congratulate you. More than half of couples experiencing such a loss don't survive as a couple.

Men and women grieve so differently. We each have a tendency to put blame, or think the other doesn't care, or isn't hurting.

Men, you've been taught men don't cry. Sometimes men distance themselves from the pain and the emotions so they don't cry. Men are the providers and protectors. In these situations, which are out of your control, you weren't able to protect your baby or your wife from this happening. Men are brought up to fix things. They cannot fix this situation, they can't undo it or redo it. Sometimes they feel so helpless, yet feel they need to be strong for their mate, especially right now. Men feel they need to make all the decisions, shield her from more pain, meanwhile pushing their own hurt away.

Once home, men tend to get busy. Busy keeps them from thinking. Often men will over indulge in work, or drink to keep from feeling and thinking.

Moms come home, sometimes their arms literally aching to hold that baby. Their bodies know they've had a baby, the breasts become engorged with milk.

A nasty reminder to mom she has no infant to feed. Mom may still have to wear maternity clothes for a little while until her body changes, but she's not pregnant. Maybe she's had a cesarean, and has no baby for it. People don't want to hear her labor story because her baby died. All these things are painful reminders of what was to be.

People who haven't heard the sad news may call and ask "Haven't you had that baby yet?" "When are you due again?" When you're out in public and people realize you're not pregnant, may ask "When did you have your baby?" "Well, what did you have?" All of this is so hard to face and answer.

While dad goes back to work, probably within a few days, maybe a week at most, mom is sitting at home, still healing from delivery. She has a lot of time on her hands. Thinking, remembering, wondering, questioning, assuming, hurting, crying, praying, sleeping, etc. are her constant companions.

Moms can become consumed with her grief. Some dads get so they dread going home because mom is so sad, teary, and emotional. He can't fix it!!! **HINT HINT:** Dad's you don't have to fix it! You do need to be there though! Just listen if nothing else. Hold her, let her cry and talk. You need the closeness, intimacy, and communication.

There have been couples who have never made love again after the loss of their baby. Women are such darn emotional creatures. Things run through our heads that keep us from being intimate: Things like, sexual intimacy is what started this whole thing. (this is how I got pregnant, because I got pregnant, I've lost this baby) **OR** how can I enjoy sex when I feel so bad or am hurting so much. Sometimes there may be an underlying issue of anger, guilt, or resentment that keeps us from intimacy.

Couples need to talk and share what each other is thinking and feeling and accept wherever the other is coming from. Grief is so different for every person and we all go through grief at different paces and stages. We must go through this valley of grief in order to heal. Healing doesn't mean forgetting.

I guarantee you will never forget this baby and life will never be the same. Anyone experiencing such losses is a changed person. I don't have answers as to why such things happen.

When you're ready though, I challenge you to do something in honor or memory of your baby that died. Books like this one come out of broken hearts to help someone else with theirs. Know that going through your labor or surgery was hard work with no reward at the end. It was a labor of love no matter how long it was, how long it lasted or how far along your pregnancy was.

Think about your time of loss. What helped you, who helped you? What things that were said hurt you? Comforted you? When you learn of someone else going through a loss, step up and be there for them.

I want to assure you that you will never forget about this pregnancy, this baby you've lost. When I interview patients in their 40's, 60's and 80's, I do ask because of my labor and delivery and bereavement back ground, "How many pregnancies did you have?"

These mom's will tell me exactly how many children they have, how many they lost, they can tell me how far along they were with the baby they lost, they can recall such detail of that time. Most elderly women, because of how things were then, were not allowed to see or hold their infants and usually they were buried without the mom's being there. I want you to know that most women who have had abortions, do not forget their lost pregnancies either.

In Isaiah 49: 15-16 it states: "Can a mother forget her little child and not have love for her own son? Yet, even if that could be, I will not forget you. I have carved your name upon my palm."

I have no doubt in my mind that all of our babies are in heaven. My concern is: What plans are you making to be sure you'll be reunited with them someday…..in heaven?

October 15th is Pregnancy and Infant Loss Remembrance Day.

If you would like a lapel pin of a child carved into Jesus' hand (Isaiah's scripture) please send $2.00 and SASE to

Helping Hands,
P.O. Box 223
Lowell, IN 46356

There is hope. I want you to know that the intense pain, aching, and emptiness will not last forever, if you walk through the valley of grief. If you deny it or remain completely consumed by it, you cannot heal. Healing comes in many forms. Healing does not mean forgetting. Healing means, that there will be a day that you will be able to laugh again and not feel guilty about it. You will be able to talk about your loved one in confidence not in tearful emotion. Healing means there will be a day when you feel life is worth living and things are going to be ok. Never the same, but ok. When you are able to reach out to someone else who is hurting, know you're healing.

Believe it or not, there will be **a day**, that you won't think of your baby. Many feel very guilty when this happens. Do not beat yourself up. As time passes, your consuming thoughts will be less. Again, you will never forget.

I hope I've been able to touch and help those of you who have read this information, bring comfort and knowledge to those who are hurting.

You are not alone.

To Helping You....From Helping Hands

Sandi RN, BSN, Bereavement Counselor

Parish Nurse

Definitions

The prefix **mis** according to Webster's dictionary means 1) wrong, wrongly, bad, badly. 2) no, not · **Carriage** is defined as 1) act of carrying, transportation. (Bearing is a synonym for carriage.) · Bearing: being a support or supporting part. The act, power or period of producing young, the ability to produce. An enduring, endurance.

v **Miscarriage** is defined by Webster as 1) a failure to carry out what was intended. 2) failure to reach it's destination 3) the expulsion of a fetus from the womb before it is sufficiently developed to survive (outside the womb) v **Pregnancy** : prefix **pre** means before. The root word **gnasci** means born. This time of carrying (enduring of a period of time) a fetus/baby refers to the time before it is born. Pregnancy is having offspring developing in the uterus (womb) Pregnancy is intended to carry the developing baby to it's final destination which is delivery at 38-40 weeks of growth in the uterus.

From Webster's point of view, when a pregnancy cannot carry its offspring to it's final destination or to term, to the developmental stage where the fetus (baby) can survive outside the womb, it is a miscarriage. A **miscarriage** is when things go wrong, badly. For whatever reason, the body is not able to carry the baby to it's full term, or age of viability (being able to survive outside the womb) to it's natural, or intended destination which is a live birth.

I feel I need to clarify some terms that we, medical personnel use, that can be confusing and maybe hurtful, although they are not intended to be. Sometimes our medical knowledge, jargon and quest for facts overrides our compassion and sensitivity.

The word abortion has many emotions and thoughts attached to it. In reality, the word **abortion means to miscarry**. It is the loss of a pregnancy, fetus, baby, at a stage when the fetus cannot survive outside the womb. Abort means to stop. With a miscarriage or abortion, the pregnancy is stopped. Abortion/miscarriage is the actual process of the passing of the fetus/baby or "products of conception" from the womb. Some of these phrases used take away the emotion and attachment to a baby.

According to J.B. Lippincott Co., "Maternal and Child Health Nursing" the term fetus, refers to the developing offspring from the 8th week after conception until birth occurs. Again, the medical field uses the term fetus all the way thru the pregnancy.

I have talked with parents, while crying their eyes out, cannot understand why their doctor told them they'd had an abortion. They didn't have their pregnancy ended, they didn't kill their baby. The physician probably said something about them having had a spontaneous abortion and abortion is all that was heard. To medical personnel: - **spontaneous abortion**: is a miscarriage. It is a miscarriage that "just happens" It was not planned, enhanced, or induced. The fetus has died. All of the components of the pregnancy were passed, or expelled from the womb. No further treatment is usually necessary. **-incomplete abortion**: The fetus has died and the body has attempted to miscarry the pregnancy. Not all of the components of the pregnancy have been passed. Some parts, have been retained in the womb (uterus) and need to have help in coming out. Usually a D & C is indicated. A **D & C** (dilation and curettage) is done to remove any remaining tissue from the pregnancy for the woman's health to protect her from hemorrhage and infection. -**missed abortion**: the pregnancy has ended, the fetus has died. There is no heartbeat, but for whatever reason, the woman's body has not acted to miscarry. Sometimes it is determined at a prenatal visit that the fetus has died, no heartbeat can be found this time. Usually an ultrasound is ordered to confirm that the fetus has died. Usually a D & C will be scheduled to prevent complications from occurring for mom's health. -**Induced abortion or therapeutic abortion**: is what most people think of when they hear the word abortion. These pregnancies are willfully, intentionally ended, abrupted, stopped. These fetuses (babies) are alive when a means is used to stop life. These abortions are done when the fetus (baby) is not capable of survival yet outside the womb. Usually before 20 weeks of pregnancy. There have been some miracle survivals!! A word of compassionate warning to anyone who has a pregnancy with severe complications. If you've been told your baby has severe birth defects or conditions that are "incompatible with life" your doctor may offer to "induce labor" at an early stage of development, or prior to the fetus/baby being full term. What would be the purpose of "inducing labor" if it would be prior to the infant being able to survive outside the womb, other than to just let it die? If your infant has known birth defects or health conditions, the womb is it's safest place. Even though emotionally it is difficult to carry/continue your pregnancy knowing there's something very wrong with your infant, and that your infant may not survive because of the complications it has, your intended job is to carry and protect that infant to it's natural destination which may or may not be full term. You and your uterus are the safe house for that fetus/infant for how ever long nature grants it. If we induce labor at an early stage and have no plans to support the fetus, provide for it, or sustain its life, it's an induced abortion. The fetus will be expelled from the womb and allowed to die if the induction method didn't kill it first. If we induce labor at an early stage for mom's health, i.e.: toxemia, pre-eclampsia, HELLP Syndrome etc, chances are, everything possible is going to be done to help the baby survive. It still may not survive if it's really premature, but the difference is the attempt to save life.

If your baby has conditions that are not compatible with life, God and the nature of life will take over. Chances are the pregnancy will not carry out to full term, chances are your baby may die before delivery or shortly after. There is no need for you to bear the guilt of inducing the death of your infant. I would encourage you, instead, to make plans, to make the most memories you can with what little time you will have. As hard as it will be emotionally, focus on the little life you're a part of for a little while. **-Partial birth/late term abortion**: Late term pregnancy is far enough along that the infant should be able to survive on it's own outside the womb. (Unless it has conditions that are incompatible with life) Partial birth means the infant in manipulated in the uterus, to be delivered feet first. These infants are alive as they are partially delivered. Abortion at this point means killing the infant before it is completely delivered. Killing the infant before it's head is delivered and breath can be taken. If the mother's health is in jeopardy and the infant needs to be delivered prior to term, this can be done without killing the baby. All measures should be taken to support this infant and help it survive a premature delivery.

If the fetus/baby has multiple birth defects or conditions stated to be incompatible with life, then nature will kick in or if doctor feels labor needs to be induced, the infant does not have to be killed to be delivered. Then the parents have a choice of "doing all that can be done to save or maintain" the life, or they can choose to simply hold that baby for what ever time they have and make as many memories as they can that will last a lifetime. Hold and treat that infant with love and dignity until it's dying breath. I wouldn't want any parent to live with the guilt of killing an infant. Sometimes, when an infant dies in the uterus before term or at term, labor may need to be induced for mom's health protection. Again, an ultrasound is done to confirm the fetus/baby has already died. It is very difficult going through labor (natural or induced) and sometimes a cesarean even, with no baby to take home when it's over. This induced labor is for mom's health precautions and the preservation of the baby's body. The big controversy is when does life begin? Are fetuses humans? I would like to leave you with a few scriptures that talk about life, life in the uterus. After reading these scriptures, you need to draw your conclusions and take a stand on what you now know about abortion. Get involved, support pro-life organizations, contact your state representatives and legislators regarding your views.

Genesis 25:21-3- fetuses struggling inside the womb
Genesis 18:10- Foretelling of a pregnancy and son
Exodus 21:22- punishment for causing a miscarriage
Leviticus 17:11- Where there is blood there is life!
Psalms 139:13-15- development of life **Ecclesiastes** 11:5- the wonder of pregnancy **Ecclesiastes** 3:2- there is time to be born **Proverbs** 31:8,9 We are to speak up for the dumb and defenseless **Isaiah** 44:2 in God's care **Isaiah** 49:1,5- divine call to the unborn **Jeremiah** 1:4,5- God's prenatal plan for Jeremiah **Isaiah** 49:15- God's promise **Matthew**

1:23- Fortelling of Mary's pregnancy, son, and his name **Luke** 1:39-44- baby's leaping at the sound of voice **Luke** 13:16,41 Foretelling of Elizabeth's pregnancy, his son and his name and his future presonality, purpose.

Grief: a normal, internalized reaction to the loss of a person, thing, or idea. Our emotional response to our loss.

Bereavement: The state of having lost something,, significant other, or significant things. Our sense of will.

Mourning: Taking the internal experience and expressing it outside of our self. The cultural expression of grief.

Traditional: Years ago families put wreaths on their doors. Black clothing was worn for a certain amount of time. Women wore black veils. **Today:** Police officers wear a black band on their arm, our country lowers flags to half-staff. Funerals and visitation are the norm.

Creative: Writing letters to the deceased. Displaying pictures of loved ones at the funeral, video of loved ones life playing at the funeral visitation, video taping of the funeral service. Releasing balloons to the deceased, planting trees or flowers in memory of a loved one, naming stars after a loved one, making shrines and crosses either at the site of the death or at the cemetery.

Rituals The behaviors we use to do our grief work.

Five Stages of Grief

1. **SHOCK AND DENIAL**
   - -I can't believe this is happening
   - -There must be a mistake
   - -You're wrong!

   Behavioral Responses to the News
   - -lack of comprehension of the situation
   - -withdrawal
   - -refusal to eat
   - -sleep disruptions
   - -create a fantasy world to deny what's real
   - -difficulty in concentrating and following directions

2. **ANGER**
   - -How dare this happen to me!
   - -Where is God when I need him?

-Why didn't God keep this from happening?

-I must have done something bad to deserve this

3. **BARGAINING**

-What do I have to do to undo this?

-Making promises to God or others that you will change, live differently, do good for others etc, if He'll just undo what's happened.

-Making irrational expectations of self to replace or undo what's taken place.

4. **DESPAIR**

Usually 4-6 months following the death or trauma. This may be when behavioral issues arise:

-increase alcohol use

-use of drugs

-suicidal tendencies

The thinking /rationalization:

My life will never be the same

I'm going crazy

I cannot go on

Denial/refusal to associate with "old" friends or places. Becoming anti-social and withdrawn.

5. **COMMEMORATING/ADJUSTING**

-Trying to make sense of this whole experience

-Searching and yearning, needing to know what really happened. Learning of details.

-Making the death meaningful. Knowing it is time to do something about it:

(write letters, make a memory album, journaling, write poems, draw pictures, get involved in an appropriate organization such as MADD, Cancer Society, Compassionate Friends etc.)

-You need to identify all that you have lost, your 1st child, your 2nd child, your son, your daughter etc., and what ever other terms you can identify your lost loved one with.

-Identifying the person you've lost VS the behavior/ illness/incident that caused your loss. Sort FACTS from FEELINGS.

-You are a changed person, never to be the same. Life will never be the same.

NO ONE will replace who has been lost. Finding an inner peace, inner place for the lost one where they can be carried forever, is an adjustment of feelings, emotions, thoughts, traditions, former teachings and a spiritual journey.

-How would you describe yourself before your loss?

-Who are you now? What's the same? What is different?

-You are still needed here? Who still needs you?

-You may need permission/peace from the absent person in order for your life to go on, to love again, laugh again.

-You may need a self-image make over.

Remembering is not living in the past, neither is wanting to talk about the past or crying about the significant person.

Recovering From Grief and Loss

Is it possible to recover from grief that's experienced by a traumatic loss? Who defines what is a traumatic loss? Is it possible we each perceive our loss as traumatic?

What does recovery mean?

-feeling better, physically, emotionally, spiritually?

-claiming your circumstances instead of your circumstances claiming your happiness.

-finding new meaning for living without the fear of future abandonment.

-being able to enjoy fond memories without having them precipitate painful feelings of loss, guilt, regret, or remorse.

-acknowledging that it is perfectly alright to feel bad from time to time and to talk about those feelings no matter how those around you may react.

-being able to forgive others when they say or do things that you know are based upon their lack of knowledge.

-One day.....realizing your ability to talk about the loss you've experienced is in fact helping another person get through their loss.

Marge Eaton writes in regards to healing and working through our grief:

"The day will come when the world seems all right to you again. You will feel safe, secure, and enjoy the people around you.

If you have grieved, you will be more patient and understand yourself and others better. You will appreciate people and life more. You will be a stronger person because of the pain you've had the courage to face."

"Coping with Death and Grief"

Unfortunately, there will be a day, probably more than one day, if we are a part of any familial or social group, that we will all be affected by the loss of someone very important, special, and close to us. Death is part of life.

It is the young, the sudden, the unexplained deaths that are the hardest to come to terms with. We never get over the loss of significant family/ friends, we learn to live with the loss. We must not ever forget the loved ones we've lost, they have helped make us who we are regardless of how long we knew or had them.

There is a large number of grievers who commit suicide, many others elect not to live. They exist... they walk, talk and breathe, but there is no life in them.

Finding Recovery is a Decision

Rick Warren sums it up well, in order for healing to happen:

-don't repress it, confess it

-don't conceal it, reveal it.

-Revealing your feeling is the beginning of healing.

It is my prayer, that while you journey through this valley of grief and loss, that your hearts may be softened and that you will experience the true *peace that passes all understanding, down in your heart* and that you will find your day and know that the world is ok again.

Resources

The Centering Corporation
www.centeringcorp.com
Pregnancy and Infant Loss
www.aplacetoremember.com/griefwww.html
Grief and Loss Resource Centre
www.rockies.net/~spirit/grief/grief.html
World Christian Resource Directory
www.missionresources.com/griefloss.html
Share, Pregnancy and Infant Loss Support Inc.
www.nationalshareoffice.com
www.CompassionateFriends.org
www.BereavedParentsUSA.org
www.AMENDgroup.com
Resolve Thru Sharing
www.bereavementservices.org
New Leaf Resources

www.newleaf-resources.com
www.helpinghandspublications.com

About the Author

S andi is a graduate of Indiana State University's School of Nursing with a Bachelor's Degree. As a Christian, Nurse, Wife, Mom, Grandma and foster parent she brings a variety of perspectives to light. She spent many years working labor and delivery and became a bereavement counselor. She does public speaking on child abuse, grief and death, foster care and health related topics entwined with scripture/christian living. She has designed "A Medical History and Health Diary" for all ages.

e-mail: sandirnbsn@sbcglobal.net

www.helpinghandspublications.com

www.ingramcontent.com/pod-product-compliance
Lightning Source LLC
Chambersburg PA
CBHW021250280526
45784CB00005B/2313